Hiking and Trekking in Virtual Reality

Extraordinary Exploration

Table of Contents

Chapter 1. Introduction

Unleash the intrepid adventurer within you without stepping outside! Dive into our Special Report: "Hiking and Trekking in Virtual Reality: Extraordinary Exploration," offering an exhilarating journey through digital landscapes that will redefine your perceptions of adventure. Leave the ordinary behind as we take you on a thrilling trek across virtual mountains, untamed forests, and unseen trails. This report isn't just about tech; it's about how tech can transform your walls into world wonders, your living rooms into lush landscapes. Whether you're a seasoned hiker or an armchair traveler, our report will turn your wildest fantasies into vivid realities. Experiences that were once out of reach can now be touched, seen, and felt, all from the comfort of your own home. So, what are you waiting for? Start your virtual voyage with us today!

Chapter 2. Embracing the Virtual Adventure: An Introduction

Technology has transformed the way we experience adventure and wanderlust. It has given us the means to bypass the need for physical travel and permits us to embark on epic journeys while remaining in the sanctuary of our own homes. The advent of virtual reality has been a game-changer in this arena, making the impossible now possible. Hiking and trekking in glorious, untamed terrains are no more a weekend luxury; it's now an everyday reality.

2.1. The Birth of a Digital Eden

Virtual reality (VR) was once a fantastical concept often portrayed in science fiction, a far-fetched technology that seemingly belonged in the distant future. Today, it has found its feet as an integral part of contemporary lives through various applications. Among these stand the realm of virtual tourism and adventure, offering the thrill of climbing snowy peaks and meandering through sun-dappled forests without leaving the living room.

No longer are the breathtaking views of the Himalayas or the exotic mysteries of the Amazon rainforest obscure experiences that demand time, money, and physical endurance. The technology weaved within VR developers' code capture, recreate, and deliver these experiences directly to our senses.

2.2. Understanding Virtual Reality

At the heart of this technological marvel is an amalgamation of complex processes calibrated to mimic the human sensory experience. Virtual Reality involves a head-mounted display, motion tracking, and occasionally handheld controllers, all integrated to offer an immersive sensory adventure. It convinces your brain that you're exploring rickety hanging bridges crossing over tumultuous rivers, or scaling the precarious ridges of the Rocky Mountains while you're comfortably nestled at home.

Enhancing the simulation, VR uses 3D computer graphics, video capture, and 360-degree photography – building an artificial environment that wraps around your vision entirely. It's this disconnection from the physical surroundings and an immersive engagement with the digital experience that truly defines VR.

2.3. Armchair Adventuring

Sitting in an armchair, you don the headset, ready to traverse across canyons and deserts of the virtual world. Each inch of your progress is tracked by sensors, creating a parallel movement in the digital environment you've slipped into. Step closer to a chasm, and it widens; look down, and you'll see the unfathomable abyss below; raise your eyes, and the distant horizon meets your gaze. All this while the armchair remains your basecamp.

Handheld controllers, haptic devices, and even VR treadmills, add another layer of realism to the experience, allowing you to interact – walk, run, grab, and feel – within your virtual surroundings.

2.4. From Attenborough to Everest

The virtual exploration space has something to offer for everyone. Enthusiasts can find themselves facing challenges straight from the world's hardest climbing trails, while nature lovers can enjoy tranquil walks amidst lush, serene landscapes. The content rich diversity spans from adrenaline-pumping adventures to tranquilizing tours.

Ever fancied shadowing Sir David Attenborough on one of his legendary expeditions? An immersive VR tour through prehistoric times alongside the maestro himself is now within reach. Or perhaps you've dreamt of conquering the Everest but dreaded the challenge? Scale the highest peak in the world without the fear of frostbite or altitude sickness, courtesy of VR.

2.5. Virtual Reality Therapy

In addition to the thrill and visual spectacle, virtual hiking and trekking have potential therapeutic benefits. Referred to as Virtual Reality Therapy (VRT), it has found its applications in physical rehabilitation and mental wellness programs, including those for veterans, older adults, and even patients with phobias or PTSD.

Immersive experiences like virtual hikes have demonstrated eliciting 'presence' – a psychological state or subjective perception where even though part of a non-physical world, one reacts as if it's real. This aspect plays a crucial role in VRT, where replicated environments help in exposure therapy and guided treatments.

In the end, it's clear that virtual reality is the key to a realm where boundaries blur between the real and the digital, the self and the avatar. So strap on your VR headset and join us in this revolution, because 'virtual' doesn't mean 'not real,' it's simply a different way of 'being real.' The world is now at your fingertips. Explore it on your terms, and leap into the extraordinary universe of virtual reality.

Chapter 3. Technology behind Virtual Reality Hiking and Trekking

The first generation of virtual reality (VR) was more about novelty than utility, considered by many to be a fad that could never recreate the magic of real-world experiences. Modern VR, however, has evolved far beyond simple games or short-lived excitement, becoming a promising platform for various sectors, including entertainment and education. Beyond this, VR has found homes in more unusual areas - one of these innovative fields is the realm of virtual hiking and trekking.

3.1. Hardware Essentials

For VR trekking, the primary tech components are the VR headset and the controllers. High-quality VR headsets, such as the Oculus Rift, HTC Vive, and Sony PlayStation VR, with their positional head tracking feature, can mimic the feeling of 'being there' in different environments - whether it's the peak of a snowy mountain or deep within a verdant forest.

Hand controllers, coupled with accurate motion tracking, allow interaction with the digital world. For instance, you can pick up a paddle in a VR canoeing scenario or reach for a tree branch in a forest. Some systems also have additional tracking for your body or even peripheral devices that you might use during your virtual exploration.

3.2. Software Mechanics

The backbone of a VR trekking experience lies in the software developed to simulate real-world environments. Precisely engineered algorithms power these simulations to recreate not only the visuals but also the sounds and physical reactions corresponding to your actions and movements in the digital environment. The underlying principle here is immersion, which relies on the accuracy and richness of the recreation.

VR uses something called 'spatial audio,' which gives a sense of direction and distance to the sound. This is essential to making the forest seem lush, the waterfall roar, and the birds tweet in the correct direction. Simulated wind resistance during a VR mountain climbers' exploration or the physical resistance of paddling a canoe can be achieved through haptic feedback devices, making the journey surprisingly real.

3.3. Procedural Generation and Terrain Building

One of the most essential components of an impressive virtual landscape is the terrain itself. Many VR hiking and trekking experiences rely on procedural generation to create an immersive landscape. The basic idea is to use an algorithm or set of rules that dictate the way features like terrain, flora, and fauna are generated on the fly. This ensures freshness and variability in each session, thereby augmenting the replay value.

But creating a convincing lush forest or a rocky mountain isn't easy. Developers need to incorporate features like elevation, landforms, hydrography, and vegetation accurately. They also need to account for natural occlusions — areas where objects block light from reaching certain parts of the scene, mimicking how light behaves in an outdoor environment. Sophisticated shading techniques are used to make the various elements look more realistic.

3.4. Inside the Virtual Trail

In addition to terrain, creating a convincing trail in VR needs careful attention to detail as well. The trail needs to be interesting and challenging, with varying difficulty levels for different users. Using mapping data, real-world trails can be scanned and then implemented within the VR environment. This combination of real and digital worlds allows users to embark on trekking and hiking adventures on actual trails from anywhere in the world.

3.5. User Experience: Balance and Comfort

The dream of a fully immersive VR trekking experience can quickly sour due to physical discomfort. VR-induced motion sickness is often a significant hurdle because the user's visual input contradicts physical perceptions of balance and movement. Great care is required in creating smooth transitions and limiting movements to those that can be comfortably replicated by a VR system.

To address this, a user-driven experience is critical to ensuring comfort. Hand controls, for example, can be implemented to allow users to take control of the pace or to stop whenever they want. Other comforts include quick cooling routines, VR displays fitted with "blue light" filters, and adjustable comfort settings to help prevent eye fatigue.

3.6. Bringing It All Together

Hiking and trekking in VR isn't just about the hardware, software, and user comfort, though these are vital components. It's about crafting a seamless experience that convinces the user they're immersed in an authentic environment, one full of adventure, exploration, and the sweet satisfaction of a journey well-traveled.

From high-end computer graphics and sound spatialization to haptic feedback devices and finely tuned balance systems, modern VR technology offers ways to recreate the great outdoors in an exciting yet comfortable way. The process may be complex, involving a careful blend of many different technologies, but the end result is clear: a trekking experience that can thrill even the most seasoned adventurer from the comfort of their own home. So, why hesitate? Strap on a headset and start exploring!

Chapter 4. Comparing Physical and Virtual Exploration: Pros and Cons

Our conception of exploration is undergoing a radical transformation due to advancements in immersive technologies like virtual reality (VR). A pursuit historically rooted in the physical world—hiking and trekking across challenging terrains—is now mimicked and amplified within a digital ecosystem. One may question: How does this analogue experience compare to its digital counterpart? This in-depth analysis aims to answer that question, investigating the pros and cons of physical versus virtual exploration.

4.1. The Lure of Physical Exploration

Physical exploration has a longstanding history. Traditionally, hiking and trekking have been preferred ways of connecting with nature, improving fitness, and fostering a sense of accomplishment. Various elements contributed to the charm of physical exploration.

Outdoor activities can yield tangible benefits. Beyond the rush of adrenaline, a physical exercise creates a harmony between the human body and mind. An ascending heartbeat, heavy breathing, and beads of sweat racing down the face are all tokens of a meaningful workout, contributing to cardiovascular health, muscular strength, and endurance. The human body physically responds and adapts to outdoor challenges, thereby triggering mental wellness and resilience.

The unpredictability inherent in nature plays a significant role in traditional exploration. Changes in weather, terrain underfoot or the sudden sighting of wildlife offer a constant element of surprise and an irreplaceable rush of fulfillment. Adventure enthusiasts find appeal in the charm of the unexpected, a marriage of thrill and danger that elevates the mundane to something remarkable.

Syncing with nature and detaching from the digital world may act as a balm to persistent elements of screen fatigue and tech burnout. By hiking and trekking, participants can disconnect to reconnect, achieving a peace that is often challenging to capture in today's frenetic lifestyles.

4.2. The Drawbacks of Physical Exploration

Despite the encompassing allure of outdoor exploration, there are deterring factors. Significant time, preparation, and a level of fitness are necessary to engage in physical trailblazing. It involves considerable planning, from route mapping, estimating travel time, and gathering gear, imposing constraints on spontaneous decisions.

Physical fitness and health condition are crucial. People with underlying health conditions, disabilities, or low fitness levels may find it difficult to partake in strenuous outdoor activities.

The risks of outdoor exploration must not be overlooked; accidents and emergencies can happen in the wilderness, making safety a constant concern. Weather changes can be abrupt and sometimes, dangerous, posing threats that can lead to perilous situations.

4.3. Pros of Virtual Reality Exploration

Virtual Reality (VR) exploration is an ascendant force in the current tech horizon, redefining our understanding of adventure and exploration. Here's a look at some of its unique selling points:

VR is widely accessible and exceptionally inclusive. It can provide immersive experiences to anyone, regardless of age, fitness level, or physical disabilities. Hence, everyone can experience hair-raising adventures and breathtaking landscapes typically accessible only to skilled adventurers.

Virtual environments don't succumb to the whims of weather, granting explorers enjoyment in all seasons and at any time of day. The absence of risks associated with real outdoor exploration makes VR a safe space for discovering unknown realms.

VR allows for instant teleportation to any location worldwide, transcending geographical limits. One can stand atop the Swiss Alps one moment and explore the dense Amazon rainforest the next - all from their living room.

4.4. Limitations of Virtual Reality Exploration

Despite its fascinating advantages, VR exploration inherits limitations. A fundamental drawback is the removal of genuine encounters with nature. VR simulates the environment but cannot duplicate the profound tactile engagement with the natural world. The smell of wet earth, the sense of wind on your skin, the taste of fresh mountain air - these are dimensions unattainable in virtual reality.

Experiencing nature via a technological lens can hollow the emotional connection, making the experience feel detached and 'manufactured.'

The technology's availability, while improving, is not yet universal. High-quality VR gear can be pricey, and not everyone has access to these systems. Furthermore, not all VR programs offer the level of detail or responsiveness that adventurers may desire.

4.5. The Final Verdict

Despite the immersive capabilities of virtual exploration, it doesn't appear to dethrone traditional physical exploration anytime soon. Both methods have their pros and cons, with each offering unique experiences. VR exploration serves as a fantastic supplement, an alternative, or an introduction to physical exploration.

By comparing the two, we realize that it's not a competition as much as it is a companionship. Virtual exploration in no way overrules the authenticity of physical exploration, nor does it intend to. Likewise, physical exploration acknowledges that the promise held by virtual reality to democratize the wilderness is an extraordinary leap.

Essentially, VR provides an opportunity for those who might normally be excluded from global exploration. If travel time, physical restrictions, or nerves hold you back, VR can offer you the thrill of adventure at your own convenience and comfort level.

Whether you prefer the raw, unaltered environment of the great outdoors, or the unencumbered, risk-free virtual exploration, the world – physical or digital – is yours to explore. The critical factor is to enjoy the journey, not just the destination.

Chapter 5. Top VR Systems for Outdoor Simulations

The dawn of Virtual Reality (VR) brought with it the infinite possibilities of creating and experiencing diverse environments from the comfort of one's home. This blessing of technology is bringing the outdoors to us, precisely for when we cannot step out! Herein, we provide a run-down of the top VR systems for outdoor simulations, analyzed based on their compatibility, affordability, comfort, immersion, and more.

5.1. Oculus Quest 2

Oculus Quest 2, an advanced all-in-one VR system, offers an exceptional balance of price and performance. Its broad field of view and high-definition graphics (1832x1920 resolution per eye) make this standalone platform a popular choice for outdoor simulation games. Quest 2 is armed with a powerful Qualcomm Snapdragon XR2 Platform processor, leading to a smoother experience and better graphics.

Accompanied by backward compatibility, nearly all games designed for the original Quest work flawlessly on the Quest 2. However, do note that this VR system requires a Facebook account for setup.

The hand-tracking feature, although available only for certain games, can significantly enhance the immersion experience. Coupled with an impressive battery life of 2-3 hours, the Oculus Quest 2 is a superior option.

Its ergonomic design elevates comfort, even during lengthy sessions. Users can further maximize their experience by investing in the fitting Elite Strap or the Elite Strap with Battery.

5.2. Playstation VR

The PlayStation VR, a strong contender in the VR market, is an excellent choice for console gamers. It offers a full VR experience with bright, flashy colors and a comfortable headset design.

Compatible with any PlayStation 4 or PlayStation 5, it has a strong lineup of games, including several top-rated outdoor simulation games.

With a display resolution of 960x1080 per eye and 100 degrees of field view, PlayStation VR trails the Oculus Quest 2 in terms of clarity and immersion. However, the Move motion controllers provide a tactile experience that can transform outdoor simulation games into realistic adventures.

Its cinematic mode allows one to enjoy non-VR games and videos in a simulated large screen for a captivating experience. A notable disadvantage is the lack of full 360-degree tracking, which the pricier higher-end headsets offer.

5.3. HTC VIVE Pro

Known for exceptional resolution and field view, HTC VIVE Pro is a premium VR headset for PC gamers. Its resolution of 1440x1600 pixels per eye and a 110-degree field of view make this VR headset one of the best for outdoor simulation games.

Features like front-facing cameras and room-scale tracking make the VR experience more immersive, providing the illusion of trekking on rocky terrains or exploring dense forests.

It is compatible with SteamVR, offering a range of simulation experiences. However, setup can be tricky, and you must have a high-end PC to enjoy them fully.

Its ergonomic design ensures comfort during extended periods of use. Additionally, the VIVE Wireless Adapter can make your experiences untethered, providing a seamless gaming journey.

5.4. Valve Index

The Valve Index headset, a product from the creators of the Steam platform, provides both robust performance and exceptional comfort. Its room-scale tracking with base stations and a 'knuckles' controller design help create engaging interaction and a deep sense of immersion.

With a resolution of 1440x1600 per eye, and up to 130 degrees viewing angle, it delivers crisp and clear visuals. The standout feature is the refresh rate, which at max 144Hz, is among the best in the industry. This high refresh rate helps reduce motion sickness and increases immersion while traversing the simulated hiking trails or seascapes.

Although expensive and requiring a high-performance PC for the best experience, the Valve Index's high precision and extraordinary responsiveness make it an ideal VR system for outdoor simulation games.

5.5. Windows Mixed Reality Headsets

Windows Mixed Reality (WMR) headsets are a collection of headsets from various manufacturers like HP, Acer, Samsung, and Lenovo.

These headsets offer diverse features and constitute a good mid-tier option for simulation games. They offer quick setup, with no need for external sensors, and a 105-110 degree field of view.

Although not all WMR headsets perform the same, they generally have good resolution, with the HP Reverb G2, for example, boasting a resolution of 2160x2160 per eye.

They are compatible with SteamVR, therefore giving access to an array of simulation experiences to enrich your repertoire of adventures.

Though VR technology is still evolving, it has made significant strides, influencing the way we experience virtual environments. Reading about such VR systems is akin to a glimpse into the future—a future teeming with immersive and transformative experiences. No matter which VR system you opt for, each one promises to enrich your life, breathe new energy into your daily routine and unlock new realms of adventurous outdoor virtual simulations. So gear up, prepare yourself, and embark on a journey that transcends the borders of your living room into an uncharted landscape of thrill and adventure.

Chapter 6. Designing Engaging Virtual Landscapes and Trails

In the realm of designing captivating virtual landscapes and trails for virtual hiking and trekking, it's important to blend technological advancement with an understanding of human behavior and psychology. Our virtual terrains aren't just about recreating photorealistic settings – we also need to create experiences that evoke emotions and tell stories. By merging technical excellence and artistic vision, we can provide hikers with an immersive experience that rivals, or even exceeds, the thrill of bodily exploration.

6.1. The Heart of Virtual Terrain Design

Designing virtual landscapes begins with acknowledging the need for a multi-disciplinary approach. Our team encompasses talent from varied fields - computer graphics, geography, geology, and even environmental psychology to create the most realistic and engaging trail designs. Rendering techniques are essential to provide ultrarealistic graphics; however, it might not be enough to captivate users. We also need to tap into the emotional and psychological nuances that landscape holds for hikers. By considering the user's experience from multiple magnitudes - from the grand vista scale to the sensory-rich, small-scale experience – we ensure that the design appeals to all types of users.

6.2. Mapping the Real to the Virtual

Virtual landscapes are often inspired by reality, meaning geographic realism is paramount. Real data sets including Digital Elevation Maps (DEMs) and lidar can be used to provide the backbone for a layout, which is subsequently overlaid with textures and lighting to give it life. To avoid instances of "uncanny valley", the right balance between realism and artistic license is vital. For instance, trees should sway subtly to evoke motion, but overdoing it can make the environment look artificial. When done correctly, users feel like they're walking in real forests or scaling actual mountains - without even stepping out of their home.

6.3. The Art and Science of Lighting

Proper lighting is the magic ingredient that brings the virtual landscape to life. It alters mood, highlights pathways, and adds depth, structure, and drama. Sunrise or sunset might be used to elicit emotion; midday brightness can add clarity and allow for color saturation; moonlight can create enchantment or suspense. Moreover, dynamic lighting changes – a transition from sunny to cloudy conditions or day to night – can further deepen the immersion.

6.4. Engaging the Senses

Sensory engagement is a significant part of a realistic experience. In addition to dynamic visuals, incorporating sound effects like the rustling of leaves, chirping of birds, gurgling of streams, or the crunch underfoot further enhance user immersion. Tactile feedback systems can simulate physical strain, the impact when climbing steps, or the feeling of wind against the skin - pushing the boundaries of realism.

6.5. Level Design and Interactive Elements

To keep users engaged, level designs need to incorporate elements of surprise and challenge. Intuitive signage and dynamic paths help guide users, but presenting options can create a sense of adventure. Decision points could lead to a serene glade or a steep, challenging terrain. Interactive elements, like wildlife or weather changes, further enhance user experience. It's important to judiciously intersperse these elements - too much can be overwhelming, while too little can be monotonous.

6.6. Emotional Journey

Immersive technology allows us to also design emotional journeys. The physiological reactions one has during a real hike – the thrill of reaching a peak, serenity when walking by a stream, or the awe of a scenic vista - can be carefully orchestrated in the virtual world. Attention to narrative design, pacing, symbolism, and metaphor forms the essence of this emotional journey.

6.7. User-Centered Feedback and Iteration

Ultimately, the best designs come through iteration and user feedback. Frequent testing can bring light to any missteps or opportunities. It's essential to remember that the user is at the center of experience design and creating an environment that responds and adapts to the user's experiences, abilities and ambitions is key to success.

Guided by these principles, we are at the threshold of creating immaculate virtual landscapes and trails that stretch the boundaries of what's perceived as possible. Just as every journey begins with a single step; every trail design begins with a spark of imagination, fostered by technological ingenuity and sanctified by the emotional resonance that each path holds for the virtual voyager.

Chapter 7. Risk, Safety, and Environmental Impact: The New Advantages

Virtual exploration's ushering in a new era of adventuring, placing a premium on risk management, user safety, and environmental conservation. Unlike traditional outdoor activities, which often carry the potential hazards of unpredictable weather, wildlife encounters, or trail injuries, virtual reality (VR) hiking and trekking eliminates these risks, enveloping users within a controlled environment where safety is paramount.

7.1. The Dawn Of Risk-Free Adventure

VR melds the thrill of the outdoors with the sanctuary of interior spaces, creating a risk-free environment for all of your adventures. This takes the unpredictability out of exploring new terrains; you no longer have to worry about possible injuries, wild animals, or weather conditions.

With VR, risks associated with altitude sickness, dehydration, and extreme weather are made obsolete. You're safe from the perils of loose footing leading to sprained ankles or worse, broken bones. It also ensures you are safeguarded against dangerous encounters with wildlife.

Users navigate their VR journeys, adapting to their comfort levels and capabilities without the factors traditional outdoor adventures impose. Furthermore, developers have crafted emergency exit protocols within the VR journey for users who might experience discomfort or dizziness, exemplifying the new world of risk-free adventuring.

7.2. Removing Physical Limitations: The Inclusion Revolution

Embodying the core principle of inclusive design, VR systems let you bridge constraints of the physical world. Regardless of the physical capability of users, VR allows everyone to become intrepid explorers.

In this virtual world, users no longer have to miss out on exciting experiences due to fear of heights or physical ailments. VR trekking and hiking take into account the varying endurance levels, ensuring exhilarating experiences for both seasoned trekkers and those who may not be physically trained for the rigors of high-altitude climbing.

7.3. Environmental Impact: Towards A Sustainable Future

Virtual adventures, while enthralling, also have a deeper meaning in terms of ecological impact. They act as instruments promoting the responsible use of our natural resources and the protection of our environment.

Every footfall on a real mountain trail has an impact. Traditional trekking can lead to trail erosion, vegetation damage, or in some instances, even disturb local wildlife. In contrast, the imprint of your virtual footstep fades away as soon as you move forward, leaving no trace behind.

VR exploration consumes only electricity, significantly reducing your carbon footprint. A journey which required air travel and fuel-guzzling SUVs is now just a few clicks away. This is optimal for environmentally-conscious explorers, creating an immersive adventure without harming the planet.

Moreover, these virtual landscapes foster a heightened sense of appreciation for the environment. The opportunity to immerse yourself in lush forests, pristine beaches, and towering mountain ranges might cultivate a more profound understanding of why these places need to be protected.

7.4. The Future Of Virtual Exploration

The impact of VR on hiking and trekking is truly transformational, blazing the trail for adventurers everywhere while prioritizing environmental conservation. The future may even hold more advantages including real-time data analysis, augmented reality integration, and the possible introduction of multi-player modes to connect the community of explorers in the virtual sphere.

In conclusion, VR offers a far-reaching vision of risk management, inclusivity, and environmental conservation. We're on the cusp of the next frontier of exploration - from your living room's safety, you can trek through virtual mountains, experience world wonders and satisfy the call of the wild with just a click!

The world is your oyster, or rather, your VR headset. Adventure has never been this safe, inclusive, and kind to our planet. So, strap in, and let the journey begin. With VR, you'll find the only risk is not wanting to return to reality.

Chapter 8. A Guided Tour of Most Popular VR Hiking and Trekking Experiences

Whether you're a VR veteran or just beginning your journey into the virtual sphere, the variety of hiking and trekking experiences available will amaze you. The hikes are realistic, immersive, and can transport you to another world. From the snowy peaks of Everest to the green meadows of the Swiss Alps, the possibilities are as open and unending as the landscapes portrayed.

8.1. The Path To VR Trekking

For anyone unfamiliar with virtual reality technology, it might seem a daunting space to explore. However, modern VR is designed to be user-friendly, intuitive, and accessible. To experience a VR hike or trek, you need a VR headset (like an Oculus Rift or HTC Vive), an application that creates the virtual environment, and a PC or console to run the application. Check the product's specifications before purchasing to ensure your device can handle the software's demands.

8.2. Oculus Rift: A Prime Mover in VR

The Oculus Rift is a popular VR headset owing to its high-resolution display and 6DOF (Degrees Of Freedom) motion tracking. Hiking and trekking enthusiasts can explore a myriad of virtual trails using the Rift.

One notable experience is 'The Climb,' a virtual rock climbing game.

Players find themselves tackling dangerous cliffs in various environments. While not a traditional hiking game, this experience offers palpable thrills and a real sense of achievement to scale the virtual heights.

8.3. HTC Vive and Its Virtual Treks

The HTC Vive, another powerful VR headset providing a high-quality, immersive experience, offers several hiking options. The most famous among them is 'Real VR Fishing', which takes you through detailed, picturesque landscapes. Despite being a fishing game by design, exploring the environments becomes a gripping adventure in and of itself.

Another robust offering for the HTC Vive is 'The Vanishing of Ethan Carter VR'. This game combines mystery, exploration, and stunning scenery to create an engaging VR hiking experience.

8.4. Virtual Reality Nature: Trails and Parks

Beyond individual games, numerous VR experiences take you on exploratory tours involving a variety of natural environments.

'National Geographic Explore VR' is one of them: it gives you the chance to kayak through icebergs, dodge falling debris, or climb a monolithic ice wall at Antarctica's face! While the focus of 'National Geographic VR' is not exclusively on hiking or trekking, it provides outdoor enthusiasts an awe-inducing experience of travel and exploration in some of the world's most stunning landscapes.

8.5. Guided VR Hiking: Healthcare and Therapy

Even in healthcare, guided virtual reality hikes are gaining momentum. They serve as an effective tool for physical therapy and mental wellness. Products like 'Rendever's VR platform' provide elder care communities with a real-world hiking experience. It replicates the activity for those who, because of health reasons, cannot go outside but still enjoy the therapeutic effects of being in nature.

8.6. More Than Just a Walk: Active VR Trekking

Virtual reality experiences are not limited to visual and aural stimulation. Products like the 'VirZoom VZ Sensor' allow users to get physically active. This add-on sensor turns your existing stationary bike into a VR-compatible device that, when synced with a VR game or app, allows you to trek or cycle through several landscapes, conjuring a complete sensory experience.

8.7. VR's Future in Hiking and Trekking

VR's potential to engage users is immense; hence, developers continue to experiment and explore more exciting experiences for users. Technological advancements could make future VR hiking and trekking experiences even more lifelike with haptic feedback and accurately replicated terrains. Till then, the prospects remain endless; there is always something new for every kind of adventurer.

Ultimately, the goal is to promote wellness and garner a deep appreciation for our natural world, virtually. The times ahead for VR hiking and trekking are promising, with a steady stream of applications vying for the attention of those seeking to conquer new, albeit virtual, terrain.

Chapter 9. Staying Fit and Active with Virtual Outdoor Exercises

Ever since the advent of Virtual Reality (VR), the boundaries of fitness and physical activity have been drastically expanded. The once heavy reliance on physical spaces such as gyms and outdoor parks has given way to a wave of indoor exercises fueled by tech-driven experiences.

Our once static living rooms have been transformed into dynamic exercise studios, with mountains to climb, rivers to cross, and trails to jog, all from the comfort of home. For fitness enthusiasts keen on maintaining a regular workout routine, or for adventurers unwilling to let a lack of time or inclement weather get in the way of their outdoor excursions, VR outdoor exercises are a game-changer.

9.1. VR and Fitness: A Winning Combination

At its core, VR is a form of immersive illusion, an artificial environment that can be so convincingly real that your mind interprets it as such, even though you are safely at home. Mid-air cliffs to scale, bottomless pits to leap over and rugged terrains to navigate stimulate your senses and push you to engage your body to 'survive' or 'excel' in these virtual scenarios, effectively creating an energetic, adventurous workout regime.

Within the realm of VR outdoor exercises, users have the ability to simulate real-life movements in a digital world, which directly contributes to their physical wellness in the real world. Walking, running, climbing, and jumping actions involve a broad range of muscle groups and help to improve strength, boost cardiovascular health, and increase flexibility.

Moreover, in this digitally-infused fitness framework, fatigue is a concept practically tossed out of the window. Since your mind is so engrossed in a virtual journey, the physical exertion seems less taxing, and you are often far less aware of the effort you're putting in until the end of your routine.

9.2. Identifying Suitable VR Activities

With a smorgasbord of VR workouts, selecting the best fit can be a process. Nearly every traditional outdoor activity has a VR counterpart today, including, jogging, mountain climbing, skiing, kayaking, and more. It is vital to identify those activities that align with your physical capabilities and your fitness objectives.

For cardiovascular enthusiasts, the equivalent of a heart-pounding run or a steep uphill climb in a VR-enabled environment can be an excellent choice. If you aim to enhance flexibility, then opt for digital adventures which would necessitate tasks such as ducking under branches or leaping over fallen logs. If it's muscle strength you're aiming for, VR climbing, with its requirement for outstretching and pulling, is ideal.

9.3. Necessary Equipment

Embracing VR for fitness goes beyond the purchase of a VR headset. To create an engaging, safe, and productive VR fitness environment, you should consider acquiring a VR-compatible treadmill or other similar devices. VR treadmills support your natural gait as you run or walk, facilitating an immersive, smooth experience.

VR controllers or gloves are also important. They track your hand

and arm movements, which then gets translated into the VR world, allowing you to push, pull or hold as you would in real-life.

Another essential would be safety mats or fitness-centered VR room dividers that can protect you from any actual accidental tumbles as you traverse your virtual landscapes.

9.4. A Tailored VR Workout Routine

Planning a fruitful workout routine would involve a combination of activities aimed at different strength building and cardiovascular objectives. Divide your routine into multiple sections including warm-up exercises, high-intensity exercises, and cool-down activities. The VR games and activities within each of these sections should evolve as your fitness level improves, pushing your boundaries further.

9.5. Wrapping Up: Staying Motivated

An interesting aspect of VR fitness that not only fosters physical health but also mental wellness, is its ability to sustain long-term interest in the workout routine. Given the gamified nature, the desire to beat high scores, unlock achievements, and discover new in-game terrains instills a sense of purpose and excitement, making each workout feel less like labor and more like leisure.

While VR is an exciting modern element that can give a fresh twist to your workout regimen, it's crucial to remember it is a tool in your fitness journey and not the entire journey itself. VR workouts should be comfortably interwoven with your overall wellness goals. Also, being aware of the limitations and safety considerations of the technology will help you make the most of this novel fitness frontier.

Utilizing the ground-breaking potential of VR we can blend the impossible with the achievable - accomplishing indomitable physical acts while being aware and respectful of our own limits. Change up your workout routine or passionately pursue your latest VR adventure knowing you're not just playing a game, you're crafting a healthier, fitter future.

Chapter 10. Social Aspects: Group Hiking in Virtual Environments

In the past, hiking enthusiasts longed for the camaraderie forged on the trails. Today, virtual reality (VR) hiking not only presents new landscapes but also an evolving social space—we'll explore how group trekking in VR revolutionizes the concept of social interaction.

10.1. The Evolution of Social Interaction in VR

Advancements in technology have expanded the applicability of VR. It isn't just about offering a single-user immersive experience anymore, but about providing a collective space where users can interact. Group hiking in VR is a fantastic example. Corresponding to real-life group hiking, VR platforms enable users to explore digitally recreated trails along with their friends, family, or even strangers from across the globe. You are not just sharing a physical space, but objectives, challenges, and triumphs in a virtual world. The shared experience fosters relationships and enhances social dynamics—an evolution in social interaction that transcends geographical boundaries.

10.2. Building Communal Experiences through Group Hiking

VR technology extends beyond the creation of lifelike environments; it also builds shared adventures. Now, hiking experiences aren't confined by physical proximity. Users worldwide can form hiking groups or join existing ones, exploring breathtaking landscapes together. This reinforms not only the social aspect of VR but also the fundamental notion of shared experiences. It encourages socializing, teamwork, and shared responsibility as users strive together to conquer virtual mountains.

10.3. Impact on User Engagement and Interaction

Group VR hiking contributes significantly to user engagement and interaction. The groups make virtual hiking more inviting and enlarge the social ambit of users who have common passions, irrespective of their actual locations. It boosts motivation: users feel more encouraged to reach goals, inspiring each other along the way. By creating interactions akin to real-life hiking, VR intensifies the overall user-engagement, resulting in a more rewarding and fulfilling experience.

10.4. Overcoming Social Barriers

Virtual environments also overcome social barriers. People with mobility issues, physical constraints, or those who live in remote areas, who were once excluded from social hiking circles, can now participate. It's a more inclusive platform, not bound by the regular constraints we face in real life.

10.5. Lessons from Virtual Group Hiking

Virtual group hiking offers many lessons that propagate beyond the realm of VR. It teaches users about the importance of cooperation, shared responsibilities, and mutual support. Virtual mountaineering endeavors instill negative capability—spurring innate resilience and endurance. Users learn to handle challenges, develop mutual respect, and realize the value of working as a team to achieve a shared goal, making the global community a bit more cohesive.

10.6. The Future of Social Hiking in VR

Looking forward, VR's social aspect will continue to grow. We'll see more personalized avatars, enhanced communication modes, haptic feedback for simulated touch, and more. Rewinding to a few years back, who would've thought that hiking with your friends from different parts of the world was possible, all while sitting at home? As technology fosters these connections and experiences, we stand on the brink of an exciting future—one where connection and participation are more accessible and inclusion is the norm.

In conclusion, the social possibilities of VR appear boundless. The group hiking experience in VR mirrors the real-world sense of community and camaraderie, while also offering an inclusive platform for those who were previously unable to participate. As VR technology advances, so too will the social experiences that it fosters, redefining the notion of a global village. We are not just spectators in this shift but active participants, pioneers exploring new societal frontiers in the realm of virtual reality.

Chapter 11. Futuristic Outlook: The Evolution of VR Hiking and Trekking

While the advent of virtual reality (VR) has primarily been witnessed in the realm of entertainment, it is increasingly making its mark in the realm of fitness and outdoor adventures. VR technology, specifically pertaining to hiking and trekking, has developed exponentially over the past few years. What once seemed like a distant fantasy has now become a tangible reality.

11.1. Rise of VR Hiking and Trekking

The initial instances of VR hiking and trekking emerged in the early 2010s. The first applications were simple, offering users a straightforward experience of exploring digital landscapes. However, they were revolutionary for their time, providing digital avatars of real-world paths and trails to be traversed in a virtual environment. Users could feel as though they were interacting with the surroundings, albeit it was quite rudimentary.

As technology progressed, so did the detail contained within these applications. Developers began to include elements such as different weather conditions, changing seasons, and the visual phenomena you would witness in real-life hiking treks, such as stunning sunsets and sunrises. In the beginning, these changes were time-bound, but as the technology and coding evolved, they became responsive to user interaction.

11.2. Integration of Tactile Feedback Systems

One significant catalyst in the evolution of VR hiking and trekking has been the integration of tactile feedback systems. These innovative systems allow users to physically feel aspects of their virtual environment. When this technology got coupled with high-resolution VR headsets, the experience got far more immersive.

A combination of haptic devices, specially designed treadmills, and controllers allow you to feel the surface you're walking on, the resistance of an incline, or even the vibration of a phone in your virtual pocket. Some developers have gone as far as to include smell in their VR experiences, embedding the scent of fresh pine or rain-soaked soil into their games.

11.3. Dynamic User Interaction

In the last three years, we've witnessed a giant leap regarding interaction mechanisms within VR for hiking and trekking. Users are no longer just passive participants, taking a linear tour through a pre-rendered environment. Today's software allows users to seamlessly deviate from established paths, enabling exploration off the beaten path, and truly express their exploratory instincts.

Moreover, VR now offers multi-player options. You could organize a virtual hike with friends or join a group trip with people from all over the world. You might find yourself trekking through the digital replicate of the Himalayas with a friend from Tokyo, talking about your favorite camping gear while watching a virtual sunrise together.

11.4. The Role of Artificial Intelligence

Artificial Intelligence (AI) has started playing increasingly prominent roles in the development of VR hiking. It helps in creating intelligent NPCs (Non-Player Characters), enhancing environmental responsiveness, and even adjusting difficulty levels based on the user's physical fitness and completion rates of previous trails.

AI is being used to develop VR systems that can learn and adapt to the user's style. Advanced machine learning algorithms collect and analyze data from prior sessions and subsequently adjust the VR experience to match individual preferences and abilities.

11.5. Health and Environmental Advancements

The application of VR in hiking and trekking has positive health implications. For people who have physical limitations or those living in spaces not conducive to trekking, these VR experiences have provided a safe and convenient avenue to stay active.

The technological advancements have also helped in conservation initiatives. Rendering accurate models of actual trails has created an option for tourism without environmental damage. Users can explore the wonders of the world without contributing to the carbon footprint caused by travel, or directly impacting delicate ecosystems.

11.6. Tomorrow's Trek

A speculative but exciting possibility is that of a full-scale, kinetic, mixed-reality setup. This involves blending the physical and digital worlds to produce new environments where physical and digital objects co-exist and interact in real-time. This will ensure an even more immersive hiking and trekking experience in VR–one where you'd feel the wind as you traverse virtual cliffs or touch virtual flora and recognize them through their texture.

As we venture into the future, VR hiking and trekking promise a continuous evolution, making our virtual adventures more immersive, intuitive, and impactful. The fusion of different technologies and creative concepts is likely to push the experiences far beyond our current expectations. From exploring the highest peaks to trekking through the age-old forests, the future of VR hiking and trekking is poised to bring what was once unreachable right into your living room.